STRESS RELIEF SECRETS REVEALED SERIES

THE ULTIMATE METHOD FOR DEALING WITH STRESS

HOW TO ELIMINATE ANXIETY, IRRITABILITY AND OTHER TYPES OF STRESS WITHOUT USING DRUGS, RELAXATION EXERCISES, OR STRESS MANAGEMENT TECHNIQUES

DOC ORMAN, M.D.

Published by:

TRO Productions, LLC

P.O. Box 768

Sparks, Maryland 21152

In association with TCK Publishing

www.TCKPublishing.com

If you believe that your symptoms or your problems are beginning to get worse as you read this book, stop reading it immediately and consult a trained health professional.

Dr. Mort Orman is a board-certified Internal Medicine physician. As a medical professional, he has successfully helped and coached people to overcome their stress and anxiety related problems for more than 30 years. However, he is not a licensed nor a practicing mental health professional. As such, each individual needs to personally assess and evaluate all suggestions and advice noted in this book.

Bottom line: you are 100% responsible for how you interpret and make use of the information in this book. So please do so wisely.

OTHER BOOKS BY DOC ORMAN

TABLE OF CONTENTS

INTRODUCTION

Are you aware there's a much better method for dealing with stress than constantly struggling to manage it?

Are you aware that the secret to using this method successfully is the very same secret for learning how to consistently win at backgammon?

This is the third in a series of self-help books under the theme "Stress Relief Secrets REVEALED." The purpose of this series is to expand your understanding of human stress—what it really is, where it comes from in your life, and what your best coping options are for dealing with it.

Unfortunately, there are many myths and misconceptions about stress (and how to cope with it) that are prevalent in our society today. Many of these myths are perpetuated by well-meaning people who are sincerely trying to help others reduce their stress.

Thus, there is an urgent need for books and other educational resources that can begin to spread more accurate and helpful information about stress to millions of individuals worldwide.

Book 1: **Stress Relief Wisdom**: *Ten Key Distinctions For A Stress-Free Life.* This first book in this series contains ten powerful distinctions to help you understand stress and reality more clearly and to enable you to have more health, happiness, and success in your life.

Book 2: **The Choice Of Paradox:** *How Opposite Thinking Can Improve Your Life And Reduce Your Stress.* This second book in the series reveals ten additional secrets for having a stress-free life, each of which requires you to choose one or more opposite ways of thinking (explained in the book) to become more successful.

Book 3: ***The Ultimate Method For Dealing With Stress:*** *How To Eliminate Anxiety, Irritability And Other Types Of Stress Without Using Drugs, Relaxation Exercises Or Stress Management Techniques.* This third book in the series introduces you to a powerful three-step method for eliminating stress that, in my opinion, is far superior to stress management. This is the method I've been using for the past 30 years to drastically reduce my own stress, both personally and professionally. It's also the same method I've taught to thousands of other people who have been very thankful for the stress relief it has enabled them to achieve.

This third book, like all the others in this series, has its own dedicated website, where you can find additional bonus material, download free reports referred to in the text, sign up to receive email notifications when future books in this series are released, and find other helpful information.

Please feel free to visit and explore this dedicated website by going to: www.theultimatemethod.com .

NOTE: Each of the books released in this series so far are "stand alone" works. Thus, it is not necessary to read either of the two preceding books to fully benefit from this one. Once you finish reading this book, however, you may want to go back and read the other two. I highly recommend this—for reasons I will explain at the end of this book—but it's completely optional.

WHY I WROTE THIS BOOK

My name is Mort (Doc) Orman, M.D. and I am a physician, author, stress coach and Founder of The Stress Mastery Academy. For the past 30 years, I've been successfully teaching people how to eliminate anger, irritability, anxiety, guilt, frustration, interpersonal conflicts, and other types of stress from their lives without having to manage it.

I've written several popular print and digital books about stress, have conducted hundreds of seminars and radio interviews, and more recently have published a number of Kindle books about stress that many readers have found very helpful. Also, I've been the official sponsor of National Stress Awareness Month every April in the U.S. since 1992.

For the first 30 years of my life, however, I was horrible at dealing with stress. I was angry, frustrated, anxious and irritable much of the time. My relationships were frequently strained, and I occasionally felt so depressed and hopeless that I believed life would never be happy for me.

My stress and anxiety got so bad after I entered medical school that I finally went into therapy. Fortunately, the medical school I attended offered free psychotherapy sessions for any student who needed them.

I continued in therapy for several years, including the rest of medical school and my three years of residency training. These weekly sessions were helpful to some degree, but I never learned to fully control my emotions nor improve my relationships to any great degree.

However, I did gain some new insights into what it means to be human, and this uncommon wisdom began to make me hungry for more.

I ended my therapy sessions shortly after opening my Internal Medicine practice. But I continued to explore other personal growth and self-improvement opportunities. These introduced me to more bits of uncommon wisdom which eventually did make a difference in my ability to deal with stress, improve my relationships, and increase my overall happiness and contentment.

After a while, I started offering stress relief seminars of my own. These were vastly different from the standard stress management seminars other stress experts were offering. They proved to be wildly successful, more so than I ever imagined, and I continued to acquire additional bits of wisdom from working intimately with so many other people.

A consistent pattern started to emerge. The more insights I gained about what it means to be human, why human beings tend to have stress, and why managing stress is not our best coping option, the less stress I began to have and the more happiness and success I was noticing in my life.

WHAT DOES ALL THIS MEAN FOR YOU?

The Ultimate Method For Dealing With Stress is about the best method for dealing with stress you will ever find.

I know this is a bold statement, but I have found it to be true—not just in my own life, but in the lives of many other people whom I've worked with during the past 30 years.

As you will soon see, this method is not new. It's been used successfully by human beings for thousands of years. In fact, you've probably used it in your own life many times before.

Thus, everyone intuitively knows about this method, but few think of it as a way to deal with their stress. There is a reason for this and it has to do with what I call the "stress management mentality" of our times.

As a physician who practiced Internal Medicine for 23 years, there are very few things I saw that caused more damage in people's lives than this popular but mistaken idea that the best way to deal with stress is to manage it. This was something I didn't understand for the first 30 years of my life (I am now 65). But once I was able to see the truth about managing stress more clearly, I was able to look back and notice all the damage this one false idea caused to me and also to many of my patients.

This is not to say that managing stress doesn't have positive, even health-enhancing benefits—because it does. It's just that as a primary strategy for dealing with stress, it takes us down a path that ultimately may cause more harm than good.

WARNING: If you are currently using stress management techniques as your primary strategy for controlling stress, do not interpret anything in this book as suggesting you should suddenly stop using these techniques. While you may eventually be able to reduce your dependency on stress management, over time, by adopting some of the alternate strategies discussed in this book, prematurely abandoning any stress management techniques that may be working for your today could cause you harm.

NEGATIVE ASPECTS OF MANAGING STRESS

Most people are completely unaware of the negative aspects of managing stress. This is not surprising, since there's a very powerful multi-billion dollar stress management industry that wants to keep you in the dark about this.

One reason I wrote this book is to "blow the whistle" on this widespread deception by clearly exposing the major drawbacks to managing stress. But this book is about much more than just debunking popular myths about stress.

The main reason I wrote this book is to introduce you to a method for reducing stress that is far superior to stress management. This method is so very good, and so highly versatile, that I truly believe it should be called "The Ultimate Method" for dealing with stress.

But because of the massive amount of stress management "propaganda" we are constantly bombarded with, most people have never learned how to apply each of the three steps in this method properly.

By reading this book, you will get a detailed introduction to this method, as well as some valuable "coaching" from me in how to begin using it successfully.

How You Can Benefit From Reading This Book

Reading this book will do several things for you:

1. It will explain why—contrary to popular belief—managing stress may not actually be good for you;
2. It will introduce you to the three-step Ultimate Method For Dealing With Stress which I have found to be much better and much more useful than stress management;
3. It will show you how this three-step method is so powerful and so versatile that it can be used to deal with any type of stress you might ever experience;
4. It will give you some initial training in how to understand and use this method correctly;
5. It will highlight certain pitfalls and challenges to using this method successfully.

What this book will **not** do for you, however, is teach you how to become a stone-cold expert at using the Ultimate Method. While you may be able to reduce or even eliminate many types of stress just from what you'll learn from this book, you may need some additional training to apply this method more broadly.

You can acquire some of this additional training from other Kindle books I have published on specific topics such as:

Overcoming negative thinking

How to end panic attacks

How to reduce anger and irritability

How to truly forgive yourself or others

Also, if you like what you learn from this book, you may want to explore some of the more advanced training programs I offer through my Stress Mastery Academy.

A New Way Of Thinking About Stress

This book will introduce you to a radically new way of thinking about stress, as well as a very new way for eliminating it that you may not have thought of before. This is a huge benefit that few other books about stress can give you.

For example, you'll discover that if you want to become the best you can be at lowering your stress, the very first thing you must do is completely eliminate the word "stress" from your vocabulary. Has anyone ever given you this advice before?

You'll also find out why the secret to learning how to win against stress is exactly the same as for learning how to win at backgammon. Has anyone ever told you this before? Probably not, but you'll soon understand why I say this.

So be forewarned—this book contains some very powerful new ideas about stress you will be hard pressed to find anywhere else.

And if you gain nothing more from reading this book other than a deep understanding of what each of the three steps in the Ultimate Method are, including how they can benefit you—both now and in the future—then I believe I will have done you a great service.

Chapter 1: Why Managing Stress May Not Be Good For You

There are six components of wellness: proper weight and diet, proper exercise, breaking the smoking habit, control of alcohol, stress management and periodic exams (Kenneth H. Cooper).

Ken Cooper, M.D. is a former Air Force Colonel who is a nationally heralded fitness and wellness expert and the father of modern aerobics. He founded The Cooper Institute in 1970 and has written more than 20 popular books on health and fitness topics.

Unfortunately, Dr. Cooper and many other experts like him are also responsible for the widespread dissemination of what I call the "stress management mentality" of our times.

This mentality, which includes a seductive mix of truths, half-truths, and flat out lies about stress, has totally dominated our thinking for decades. It's so pervasive and so overpowering that anyone who dares to question any of its key components is quickly labeled a fool.

Most people have bought into this stress management mentality today—hook, line and sinker. The vast majority of my physician colleagues, including Dr. Cooper, also positively endorse it. The media perpetuates it constantly. And every member of the multi-billion dollar stress management industry, who profits from sales of books, audiotapes, seminars, and other similar "educational materials," also wants you to believe in it wholeheartedly.

Yet there are others who have courageously dared to question some of the fundamental assumptions this mentality is built upon. Some have even started to openly challenge the whole mindset publicly. I've been one of these "voices" for more than 30 years now, and I am not alone. Others have expressed similar concerns and cautions.

Consider the following quote from Richard Ecker, author of the 1985 book titled *The Stress Myth*:

"We like to believe that stress is inevitable—that life is so much more complex these days, that we are being dragged along by a runaway world which offers us less and less that we can depend on. But this belief is nothing but a myth, a myth that is at the core of the stress problem...This myth...has done more to perpetuate unwanted stress in our society than any other single factor. Ironically, the main proponents of this myth are the very ones who claim to be teaching people how to deal with stress."

THREE BASIC COPING OPTIONS

As human beings, we all struggle with stress from time to time. Whether it's emotional stress (feeling angry, frustrated, anxious, etc.), or whether it's relationship tensions, work-related pressures, stress-related physical problems, financial concerns, or anything else—we only have three basic options for dealing with these common challenges (other than simply ignoring or denying them):

The Band-Aid Approach

The Stress Management Approach

The Ultimate Approach

The Band-Aid Approach

We make use of this approach when we turn to alcohol, prescription drugs, recreational drugs, cigarettes, food, sex, shopping or anything else to quickly relieve unpleasant symptoms of stress. In the short-run, these popular coping strategies "work" very well, since they can quickly relieve much of the physical or emotional pain we may be experiencing.

However, in the long-run these coping strategies can lead to health problems, addictions, accidents, and many other harmful consequences. Thus, they are not ideal solutions for dealing with stress.

The Stress Management Approach

Our second option is to turn to a group of strategies and techniques collectively known as "stress management." These include things like yoga, relaxation exercises, meditation, biofeedback, listening to soft music, regular physical exercise, dietary changes, getting massages, taking frequent vacations, etc.

All of these strategies have many positive and in some cases health-enhancing benefits. In addition, they avoid many of the negative consequences of using alcohol, drugs, overeating, and other chemical coping methods.

However, despite their many positive benefits, using stress management techniques also has negative consequences which can outweigh most of their positive effects. If you don't already know about these *major drawbacks to managing stress*, you'll learn all about ten of them in the first two chapters of this book.

The Ultimate Approach

The third coping option is what I consider the "ultimate approach." This is knowing how to make your stress quickly and naturally disappear without using drugs, relaxation exercises or other time-consuming stress management techniques.

Most people don't know that this third approach is always available to them. Even worse, few people actually know how to use it successfully.

This ultimate approach is not only extremely powerful—it is highly versatile as well. You can use it to deal with virtually any type of stress you might ever encounter. In addition, it can also:

Improve your interpersonal relationships

Increase your overall happiness

Increase your productivity

Raise your self-confidence and self-esteem

And much, much more.

MANAGING STRESS IS NOT ALL IT'S PROMISED TO BE

The key message of this book is that *managing stress is not your best coping option*. There's another excellent method—the Ultimate Method—that is much more powerful and far more beneficial.

But you probably haven't heard about this excellent method before. And the primary reason is because of the constant drone of stress management advice that you are bombarded with every day. This dominating flow of mixed truths and untruths about stress either keeps you from hearing about this alternate method at all, or it causes you to instantly dismiss it because it doesn't fit with everything else about stress that you and others have been taught to believe.

THE NEGATIVE SIDE OF MANAGING STRESS

Whether you know it or not, there are negatives as well as positives to managing stress. You may be inclined to think the positives far outweigh the negatives. But in my opinion, if the truth was more widely known, most people would agree that it's actually the other way around.

You probably already know about many of the negative aspects of managing stress. Yet because of all the positive stress management propaganda that's been firmly cemented into your mind, you aren't allowed to think about the negatives nor discuss any contrary opinions in public.

But this doesn't change the fact that negatives to managing stress clearly do exist. And in this chapter and the one that follows it, I'm going to show you some of the most important ones.

10 GOOD REASONS WHY YOU SHOULDN'T MANAGE YOUR STRESS

To help you better understand the key weaknesses, disadvantages, and limitations of managing stress, here are ten good reasons why you might want to reconsider the wisdom of this popular coping strategy.

NOTE: If you've already read some of my other books about stress, you may have seen these ten reasons before. Even so, it's good to refresh your memory by reading them once again.

1. TIME-CONSUMING

Most stress management techniques require you to take valuable time away from your busy schedule every day. Some even require you to devote 15-30 minutes two or three times each day to be effective.

Many people who are stressed, however, may be too busy to devote 15-30 minutes two or three times a day to use relaxation exercises or other stress management techniques. Hence, time constraints are one big drawback of trying to manage your stress.

2. COMMITMENT AND DISCIPLINE

To be most effective at relieving stress, techniques such as physical exercise, meditation, yoga, relaxation, and others must be practiced continuously over long periods of time. This requires a very high level of personal commitment and discipline, which many people lack.

Even if you start out well, with high hopes and very strong intentions, your commitment to continue practicing these daily techniques may wane after a while. Thus, the need for long-term commitment and discipline is another major drawback to managing stress.

3. LIMITED BENEFITS

Even when people do use stress management techniques on a daily, consistent basis, they often find that these techniques are not very good for dealing with certain types of stressful problems. In other words, they can be limited in both the scope and depth of benefits they can afford you.

For example, stress management isn't very helpful for dealing with problems such as the death of a loved one or the loss of one's job. It's also not very good for dealing with ongoing relationship conflicts, financial stress, chronic worry, and many other common stressful problems.

If you are having major problems with your marriage, for instance, you can run 5 miles every day or punch a punching bag until you are physically exhausted, or listen to all the relaxing music you want. But will any of this fix your relationship? Mostly, the answer is no.

Therefore, when big or persistent stressful problems occur, managing stress may not bring you all the relief you want.

4. SHORT-LIVED BENEFITS

Another major drawback of managing stress is that even when this approach gives you the immediate relief you want, this benefit is often short-lived. After a while, your stress will likely come back and you'll have the same need for managing it that you did before.

This is part of the reason why many stress management techniques need to be used several times each day, every day of the year, for the rest of your life. Your stress never completely goes away, so when you exert efforts to reduce it, as soon as you stop applying these techniques, your stress quickly reappears.

5. DOESN'T RESOLVE PROBLEMS

One of the most important drawbacks of managing stress (to be discussed in greater depth in Chapter 2) is that it rarely ends your stress problems definitively. Thus, no matter how hard you work at it, or how good you become at managing stress, your underlying stress problems will continue to bother you.

Anyone who looks at this drawback honestly will have to conclude that it leaves much to be desired. However, when we are feeling stressed, and when we are struggling just to keep our head above water, we rarely notice how horribly flawed this popular coping strategy really is.

6. LITTLE SELF-EMPOWERMENT

In addition, stress management techniques such as physical exercise, relaxation, listening to soft music, or taking frequent vacations generally do little to improve our knowledge about life or our self-awareness. Thus, they do little to empower us to deal with our problems and challenges more effectively.

There are some stress management techniques, however, such as certain types of meditation, which do seem to have a dual benefit. While providing relief of our stress in the form of relaxation, they also help "retrain" our minds and expand our conscious awareness, so we may reduce the overall amount of stress we may be generating in our lives.

However, even dual-purpose techniques such as meditation often don't end up empowering us to deal with our stress as much as we would like (and as much as we are truly capable of).

7. STOPS EXPLORATION

Another drawback to managing stress is that this coping strategy keeps us from searching for—and discovering— even better ways of dealing with stress.

This same drawback occurs when people rely upon drugs, alcohol, food, or other chemical coping methods to deal with their stress. Since these methods appear to "work" in the short run, many people end up relying upon them primarily, instead of continuing to search for better and healthier ways to deal with their stressful problems.

8. CREATES DEPENDENCY

As with less healthy coping strategies, such as using drugs, alcohol, overeating, etc., the more we rely upon stress management techniques, the more we become dependent upon them. In some ways, becoming dependent upon healthy stress management techniques may be good for us.

However, since they pretty much guarantee that our stress will keep reoccurring, they can have damaging effects as well. We'll see more about why this is so in the next chapter (Chapter 2).

9. PERPETUATES MYTHS AND MISCONCEPTIONS

Another huge problem with managing stress is that it promotes additional myths, misconceptions, and other false ideas about stress that are also very damaging to millions of individuals.

In order to remain an advocate of stress management, not only do you have to force yourself to deny all of the drawbacks and limitations noted above (including the biggest one yet to be discussed in Chapter 2), but you also have to endorse many other myths and misconceptions about stress that are required to justify this flawed approach.

In addition to perpetuating the myth that the best way to deal with our stress is to manage it, stress management proponents also encourage us to believe in other popular myths about stress, such as:

Stress is an unavoidable, inevitable part of modern life.

Stress is the inappropriate activation of our body's ancient "flight or fight" response.

The primary causes of our stress are mostly beyond our direct personal control.

If you believe in any (or all) of these widespread false beliefs, you have become a victim of what I call the "stress management mentality" of our times.

Remaining trapped within this false mentality makes it difficult for you to question the prevailing dogma about stress. It also makes it difficult for you to recognize that there are better ways to cope with your stress than simply learning how to managing it.

10. THE BIGGEST DRAWBACK TO MANAGING STRESS

Now if these first nine reasons for questioning the wisdom of managing stress weren't convincing enough, there is a tenth giant drawback that dwarfs all the others.

This one giant weakness is the main reason why I believe managing stress is **not** your best coping option. I'll discuss this tenth important reason—all by itself—in Chapter 2.

CHAPTER 2: THE BIGGEST DRAWBACK OF MANAGING STRESS

One of the symptoms of an approaching nervous breakdown is the belief that one's work is terribly important. (Bertrand Russell...actually talking about causes!)

If the first nine drawbacks to managing stress aren't bad enough, there's a tenth one which is one whopper of a disadvantage.

SYMPTOMS—NOT CAUSES!

This major weakness is that, with few exceptions, stress management techniques deal **only with the symptoms** of your problems. They don't help you identify or deal with the **underlying causes** of your day-to-day difficulties.

In my opinion, this is the most costly drawback of managing stress.

Think about it for a moment—if the **engine warning light** on the dashboard of your car suddenly started flashing, would you ask your mechanic to disconnect the wire to the bulb?

Of course you wouldn't. But this is exactly what you are doing when you focus only on reducing just the symptoms of your stress.

Wouldn't you be much better off if you were able to identify and then deal with the **underlying causes** of your stressful problems in life? After all, when all we do is deal with just the symptoms of our problems, these problems rarely get resolved. This means our stress will keep coming back, over and over again.

This one giant drawback alone should make you perk up and think twice (or more times, if needed) about relying upon stress management as your primary coping strategy.

"Can't Do Much About The Causes Of My Stress"

You might be thinking that while it is makes perfect sense to preferentially deal with the causes of your stress, there's not much you can do about most of these causes.

Au contraire, my friend.

There's a heck of lot you can do about the causes of your stress, provided you understand these causes correctly.

You see, whenever we are suffering from stress, there will always be two different types of causes involved.

One type is the *external* causes we encounter. This includes external events, the behavior of other people, demands placed upon us by others, the fixed amount of hours in a day, the weather, traffic jams, the job you have, the job you lost, etc.

The other type of causes is *internal*, not external. These include our internal thoughts, opinions, beliefs, attitudes, assumptions, perceptions, values, morals, habits, behaviors, etc.

And while it may be absolutely true that you may have little or no direct personal control over many of the external causes of your stress, you always have 100% control over your own internal causes. Yet most people don't know that they have this control, and even fewer know how to exercise it consistently.

Why do so many people fail to take advantage of this incredible power they already possess to influence the internal causes of their stress?

There are two answers to this question. The first is that our social conditioning encourages us to only focus on external causes, as if internal causes don't exist. This is what the media does. It's also what many of our friends and family do. And it's also a big part of the pervasive (and destructive) stress management mentality of our times.

The second reason is that we simply haven't been taught how to correctly identify the internal causes of our stress. We aren't taught these important skills in our primary education. We rarely get exposed to them in college. And I can tell you they were never taught to me in medical school, in my three years of medical residency, or in any other of my professional training.

You Don't Have To Be A Psychologist

Interestingly, you don't have to become a psychologist, psychiatrist or any other type of mental health professional in order to understand the most common internal causes of your stress. These causes are not complex, nor are they difficult to understand (you'll see this for yourself later in Chapter 6).

They are often very simple *thought patterns* or *behavior patterns* that frequently get triggered within us. They are habits of thinking, habits of perceiving, and habits of behaving (including actions we habitually fail to take) that become part of how we "automatically" tend to react and respond to all sorts of external events in our lives.

For example, say your habit is to wake up each morning, get into your car and drive off to work without checking the radio, your cell phone or your computer for recently reported traffic problems. Then one morning, you get stuck in a horrible traffic jam that takes several hours to clear and causes you a great deal of stress.

Did the traffic jam (external circumstance) alone cause you to experience stress? No, because in this day and age you could have easily learned about this traffic jam in advance and avoided it (in most cases). So your habit of not checking available sources (internal cause) was partly responsible as well. In this example, it was a combination of both internal *and* external causes—and this is almost always the case with every type of stress we encounter.

Here's another example to further illustrate this point. You hire a contractor to do some repair work on your home. You select this contractor from all the others because his rates were the lowest and because he was nice to you and looked very honest. He then asked you for a 50% deposit to begin the job, took your money and went on the lamb.

This was horrible behavior on his part for sure, and probably very stressful for you. But was it just the bad behavior of this contractor that caused you to get scammed? Or did your own internal assumptions about his honesty, your feelings about how nice he was to you, and your lack of checking him out more thoroughly (all internal causes) play prominent causative roles as well?

And while you may not have been able to do anything to change his morals, you could have taken control of your own internal causes, which might have kept this from happening.

It's not hard to recognize and then deal with these types of internal causes. It's just that we haven't been encouraged to do this. And we haven't been taught how to most powerfully benefit from this approach.

Instead, we've been taught to take all of our problems and lump them into one proverbial basket called "stress." Then, we are advised that the best thing we can do to protect our health is to learn how to manage just the symptoms of this basket of problems.

On the other hand, if your goal is to get at the root causes of your stressful problems in life, then *stress management will never get you there.* This is because different problems often have very different causes. So you can't just lump all your stressful problems together and then try to deal with them as a group.

You've got to split them out, one by one, and examine the root causes of each problem individually. This, as I'm sure you can appreciate, is the exact antithesis of stress management.

So are you ready now to learn how to use the Ultimate Method? In the next few chapters, I'll provide you with a detailed overview.

Chapter 3: The Ultimate Method For Dealing With Stress

Teaching to unsuspecting youngsters the effective use of formal methods is one of the joys of life because it is so extremely rewarding. (Edsger Dijkstra)

So What's The Alternative To Managing Stress?

There is a powerful alternative to managing stress. Quite simply, it is to make your stress naturally go away (or reduce it significantly) *by correctly identifying and addressing underlying causes.*

This is what people who are skilled at reducing stress know how to do. It's also what you can learn how to do, if you are truly interested.

You Can Learn To Win Against Stress!

This may be hard to believe, but you can absolutely learn how to win against stress. You can learn to make most of the stress in your life naturally disappear, without having to use cigarettes, alcohol, illegal drugs, overeating, relaxation, avoidance strategies, or any other time-consuming stress management techniques.

I've learned to do this myself, and I've also spent the past 30 years successfully teaching these same stress mastery skills to others.

The Ultimate Method Explained

The method I am about to recommend to you in this book is not difficult to understand. In fact, you already know what it is. You're just not accustomed to thinking about it as a way to deal with your stress. It's actually been around for thousands of years. In fact, I'm sure you've used it successfully in your own life, many times before.

Here's what the method is in a nutshell:

The very best method for dealing with any **stressful problem** or problems in life is to:

Identify each problem <u>specifically</u>;

Identify the main <u>causes</u> of each problem;

<u>Deal</u> with the causes effectively until your problem lessens or completely goes away.

Human beings have been using this three-step, problem-solving method throughout all of our recorded (and unrecorded) history.

But we don't think to use it when we're trying to cope with our stress, and that's a shame. Because it works very well, and because you can apply it virtually anywhere—to any stressful situation you might have—now or in the future.

Granted, some underlying causes (mostly the external ones) may not be under your direct personal control, and others may not be easy for you to identify.

But when you are able to identify the main underlying causes accurately, and when they are actually under your direct personal control, you can then take steps to correct them. And if you do this, your problems will almost always get better or even go away entirely.

You Can Learn To Use This Ultimate Method Successfully

Wouldn't you love to know how use this simple three-step coping method successfully to eliminate any type of stress in your life, quickly and easily, without having to manage it?

You may think this is impossible, but it's not.

Now that you know what the three steps in this method are, it's time for you to learn how to better understand and successfully apply each one.

Let's start by looking more closely at the first critically important step in the method.

FIRST STEP: GET MORE SPECIFIC

If you want to deal with underlying causes of your "stress," many of which may be internal (i.e., within you), the first thing you need to do is train yourself to **get more specific**.

Instead of thinking that your problem is "stress," the first thing you'll want to do is *eliminate this word entirely from your vocabulary*. This will force you to get much more specific about whatever problem or problems may be troubling you. For instance:

Are you getting angry all the time?

Are you feeling frustrated?

Are you having difficulty getting to sleep or staying asleep?

Are you having physical or health problems?

Family problems?

Social problems?

Academic problems?

Substance abuse problems?

Money problems?

Self-esteem problems?

Self-Confidence problems?

Other problems?

This is an absolutely **critical first step** in the method.

WHY DO YOU NEED TO GET MORE SPECIFIC?
The reason is because specific **problems** always have very specific **causes**.

Once you become good at identifying these causes (many of which are hidden from your view), you'll be able to make most types of "stress" in your life quickly disappear, without needing to use drugs, relaxation exercises, or other time-consuming stress management techniques.

ANGER MANAGEMENT OR ANGER MASTERY?
For example, say you are getting angry or feeling irritable multiple times each week. If all you wanted to do was manage just the symptoms of this type of "stress," you could take up jogging, install a punching bag in your home, try deep breathing or use other relaxation techniques.

But if you want to get at the root causes of this problem, the first thing you must do is recognize that your real problem is **anger**. Of course, you could be having other problems contributing to your stress as well. But for now, let's just focus on this one anger problem.

Ok. So what are the causes of your anger? Why are you getting angry about things that most other people don't get angry about? And why are you getting angry so many times each week, when most of your friends, family members and peers only get angry every once in a while?

To answer these questions, you must first be able to identify all the important causes of your anger (Step 2 in the method). This includes both the external (obvious) causes and also the internal (hidden within you) causes. Unless you have all of these causes on the table, you're not going to be able to keep your anger from frequently reoccurring.

However, once you do know how to identify the specific internal causes of human anger, along with all the external causes you can easily see, you will have many more options for reducing your angry feelings than you currently believe are available to you.

For example, once you know how to specifically identify the main internal causes of human anger, you can literally make your anger quickly disappear—anytime you want! This comes from skillfully applying Step 3 in the method, and it's not very hard to do—once you correctly identify all the key hidden causes.

Once you learn about the hidden causes of anger and get good at recognizing them within yourself (as well as within others), you'll begin to notice that you aren't getting angry as often or as easily as before. This is because your understanding of human anger will have been permanently improved. As a result, you'll start having very different views of things that go on around you every day. And when you begin to look at things from your newly gained perspective on anger, certain things that made you very angry in the past may not continue to make you angry anymore!

I know this is a very simplified, high-level overview of the method in very general terms. But don't worry, I'll give you more details about each of these steps later on. I just wanted to give you a quick peak at the full method before I begin to explain it more deeply.

NOTE: In Chapter 8, the final chapter of this book, I'll show you how you can easily learn about the internal causes of anger.

You'll Be Amazed How Powerful This Method Is!

As I'm sure you can agree, the very best way to cope with any problem in life is NOT to manage its symptoms alone, but rather to identify and deal with its underlying causes.

I've spent the past 30 years teaching people how to accomplish each of the three steps in this Ultimate Method. And the results people have achieved, once they learn how to do this, are truly remarkable.

Most people today, however, including most highly-educated college graduates, find it very difficult to cope with stress in this way. Not because they lack the ability to do so, but simply because **they haven't been trained** to deal with stress in this fashion.

Chapter 4: Correctly Identifying Your Problems Is Not Always Easy

He who seeks for methods without having a definite problem in mind seeks in the most part in vain. (David Hilbert)

While you may think that identifying your problems is not a difficult task—after all you are the one having them so you should know what they are—this first step in the Ultimate Method is not always easy to accomplish.

The reason for this is that we don't have a ton of experience trying to separate and define our problems precisely. We've actually become pretty "sloppy" about how we think about our problems, because nobody demands precision from us and because we simply haven't been focused on causes, so there's no perceived penalty for being imprecise.

However, once you enter the "let's deal with causes" game, everything changes. You can only win this game if you start off by defining your problems correctly.

Paul's Story

Let me give you a real-life example to demonstrate this point. When I was in medical practice, some of my physician colleagues would occasionally refer patients to me for help with reducing their stress. One of these patients was a 36-year-old management executive named Paul, whom I wrote about in my book *The 14 Day Stress Cure* (pp. 8-9).

Paul came to see me having already defined his problem as "stress." Without even talking to him, I already knew he was defining his problem incorrectly.

In our first session together, he began by telling me about his problem called "stress." Here's how part of that initial conversation went:

Paul: I've been under a great deal of stress lately.

Me: Can you tell me what you mean by "being under stress?"

Paul: Well, I've recently been transferred to a new department and my boss is riding me pretty hard. I've got many new responsibilities and not enough time to learn how to handle them all.

Me: Is there anything else going on that makes you say you are under stress?

Paul: Yes, I'm not sleeping very well and I've become overly preoccupied with my performance at work. I felt confident and secure in my old position, but now I don't have any self-confidence at all. I'm worried that if I don't increase my productivity, I'm going to get fired.

Me: Anything else?

Paul: No, that's it. Oh, yes, there's one more thing. I've been so concerned about work lately that my sex drive has diminished, and my wife is beginning to pressure me.

Notice how Paul had lumped all of his problems together into one big basket called "stress" and that he lacked clarity, specificity and individualized problem focus as a consequence.

If Paul had known about the Ultimate Method, however, he would have rejected the word "stress" and focused instead on the first step in this method. He then could have seen that he was actually suffering from at least *seven* very specific problems:

A relationship conflict with his new boss;

Adjusting to new job responsibilities;

Poor sleep;

Loss of self-confidence;

Fear of being fired;

Reduced sexual desire;

Increasing pressure from his wife.

So instead of treating Paul with medications, relaxation exercises, or getting him to practice other stress management techniques, my first goal was to help him give up trying to deal with "stress" per se and focus instead on each of the specific problems he was having.

Once he did this, we were able to identify the main underlying causes for each of his seven problems individually. When he could see these causes more clearly, especially some of the internal ones he hadn't noticed before, he was able to take actions and make corrections that improved each problem dramatically.

SPECIFIC EMOTIONS CAN BE DIFFICULT TO PINPOINT

Our emotions, especially negative emotions such as anger, guilt, fear, sadness, worry, frustration, and others are another very common type of "stress." Once again, if you are not trying to identify the specific causes of your emotions, you can call them whatever you want. You can also mix them up and not distinguish them specifically.

However, if you want to examine the internal causes of your emotions, you've got to "diagnose" them precisely or you'll never achieve your goal.

This task can be quite challenging for several reasons. First, we're not very good at distinguishing our emotions precisely, so we haven't had much practice doing this.

Second, different people experience emotions differently. Some people, for example, know when they are feeling angry. Others may have learned to block out feelings of anger, so their awareness of when they are angry might be little or none at all.

Third, our emotions don't always occur as nice, discrete, neatly separated experiences. Human emotions are frequently "messy," meaning that multiple different emotions can sometimes descend upon us simultaneously.

Also one emotion can quickly trigger another to appear, and this second emotion can then lead to a third. When this type of "emotional chain reaction" happens, all we know is that we are feeling "upset" without precisely understanding which emotion came first, which followed next, and which was last in the chain.

For example, you may have an angry outburst one day that hurt someone's feelings. The instant you notice this, you feel guilty for what you did and then worried that you may have damaged the relationship. This all may have happened so fast that you probably didn't appreciate that three separate emotions were involved.

Each of these specific emotions—anger, guilt, and worry—all have distinct and different underlying causes. So if you wanted to use the Ultimate Method to deal with this incident, you would have to pick one or two specific emotions to focus on and then follow the next two steps in the method for each.

So you see, completing the first step in the Ultimate Method is not always easy. However, assuming that you completed this first step successfully, it's now time to select one of the problems you've correctly defined in order to tease out all of its important underlying causes.

This is the second step in the Ultimate Method, and it requires specialized knowledge and skills most people lack. These skills can be acquired, however, but there's a huge obstacle to overcome in doing so. If you don't know about this obstacle, your efforts to accomplish this all important second step are likely to go unrewarded.

Fortunately, you can learn how to overcome this obstacle by understanding what it takes to become an excellent backgammon player. I'll explain what I mean by this mysterious relationship in the very next Chapter.

Chapter 5: The Secret To Winning Against Stress

How can a 5000-year-old board game like backgammon contain the secret to having a stress-free life today? (Doc Orman, M.D.)

This chapter is not really about backgammon. It's about how backgammon embodies a key secret to mastering life that is at the heart of the Ultimate Method.

NOTE: This life-mastery principle is not exclusive to backgammon. I could have used other games or endeavors in life to demonstrate it equally well. So you don't have to know anything about backgammon—or have any interest in the game at all—in order to benefit from reading this chapter. I just chose backgammon because I had a dramatic personal breakthrough with this game that I can use to explain this key principle to you in a clear and easy to grasp way.

What In The World Does Backgammon Have To Do With Stress?

At first glance, it appears that backgammon has little, if anything, to do with relieving our modern-day stress. After all, this ancient board game is more than 5000 years old, and many people alive today have never even played it.

Besides, thousands of years ago when the game was first invented, there were no cell phones, no computers, no traffic jams, no junk food, no corporate bureaucracies or governmental red tape, no IRS, and none of the many other stressful circumstances we commonly experience today in the twenty-first century.

In this chapter, however, I'm going to reveal to you a very deep connection between backgammon and human stress which most people are totally unaware of. You see, I'm all about winning against stress, not endlessly spinning your wheels constantly trying to manage it.

As luck would have it, the most important principle for winning against stress turns out to be the very same principle for winning at backgammon. So even though stress and backgammon appear to have little in common, this 5000-year-old board game contains an extremely important secret that literally can change your life.

Now, if backgammon can actually show you how to become a winner against stress, think of all the benefits this could bring you. Your happiness and self-confidence would skyrocket. Your relationships would improve. Your immune system would be stronger. And your ability to be successful at anything you set your mind to would be greatly enhanced.

And all you have to do to get these awesome benefits is grasp this deeper relationship between backgammon and stress which I'm going to reveal to you in just a few moments.

As I mentioned earlier in this book, I may be an accomplished stress expert now, but I wasn't always this way. In fact, for the first 30 years of my life, I was a "double loser" with regard to both stress and backgammon. I didn't have a clue how to win either of these two "games." And I remained a "double loser" until I discovered the age-old secret that backgammon (and many other games) contains.

So if you'll indulge me just a bit, I'd like to tell you an illustrative story about my own personal experiences with backgammon. And while I'm telling you this story, you're probably going to think it has little to do with you. But by the time I'm done, I think you'll agree that it truly does—in a very big and important way.

MY OWN PERSONAL STRUGGLE WITH BACKGAMMON

Regarding to my own personal history with backgammon, I never even saw this game being played until I was in my late 20's. None of my childhood friends ever played the game, and to my knowledge, nobody in my family—mother, father, sister, or any of my relatives—ever played it either.

The only thing I knew about backgammon was that it had something to do with those odd-looking, pointy triangles on the flip side of every Checkers board I ever owned. But I had no idea what actually transpired in this mysterious triangular world "down under." As a result, during my early childhood and adult years, backgammon was totally irrelevant to me.

THEN EVERYTHING SUDDENLY CHANGED

When I was in my late 20's, however, I was introduced to backgammon purely by accident.

Shortly after finishing my medical residency in Baltimore, I went into private practice on my own. I also decided to take up the sport of tennis. So I joined an indoor tennis club and began taking weekly lessons from one of two tennis pros who worked full-time at this club.

These two tennis pros, named John and Jimmy, were very good friends. They were also very accomplished tennis players, and they enjoyed competing against each other every chance they got.

When their teaching schedules were light, and when they weren't playing a tennis match against each other, they would sometimes continue their competitive rivalry by playing backgammon.

I remember the first few times I observed them playing a heated game of backgammon. They always had money at stake, and sometimes a good bit of cash would change hands.

A Simple Game Of Chance

This was the first time I had ever seen the game of backgammon being played. And while I didn't understand all the rules and strategies, my first impression was that it was a pretty simple game of chance.

There didn't appear to be much skill or talent to it at all. Whoever got hot and rolled the higher dice numbers was likely to end up the winner. Or, whoever got lucky and rolled a specific number allowing them to "hit" one of their opponents unprotected pieces, thereby sending it all the way back to "go," was also likely to be victorious.

It sure looked to me like backgammon was 95% luck and only 5% skill. That is, until I started playing it myself...for money.

Getting Your "Ass-umptions" Handed To You

One day, I happened to be relaxing at the club when one of the two pros was giving a lesson and the other was free with idle time on his hands. This pro (I don't recall if it was John or Jimmy) spotted me hanging around and invited me to play some backgammon with him. I reluctantly accepted, and we played just for fun while he taught me the basic rules of the game.

Once again, it seemed like a pretty simple game of chance to me. As I got more familiar with it, I started filling in as a backgammon partner for both of these two pros on a more frequent basis.

Then, one day one of them asked me if I was ready to play for money. Like an unassuming lamb being lovingly led to its slaughter, I foolishly agreed.

Immediately, I started losing every game we played. The more I lost, the more confident I became that luck would eventually turn my way. After all, in a game that's 95% chance and only 5% skill, you're eventually going to win some of the times. Right?

As my losses continued, however, I became more and more frustrated and angry with myself. It wasn't so much the money I was losing (it wasn't all that much). Rather it was consistently losing at such a stupid game of chance that really began to gall me.

TURNING IT ALL AROUND

As time went on, and my losses and frustrations mounted, something happened one day that turned my backgammon future—and my entire life for that matter—completely around.

I finally figured out exactly why I was consistently losing at backgammon. And from that moment on, I was determined to become a winner.

Within a month or so, I was holding my own against both of these more experienced tennis pros, and I occasionally emerged as the victor. A couple of months later, I was winning consistently, much to the surprise of my two more accomplished opponents.

Over time, I developed into an outstanding backgammon player. I haven't played much during the past few years, due to other interests and passions, but when I was playing regularly back then, I was scary good.

I could even defeat most backgammon computer programs, winning on average 7-8 times out of 10. And if you were a novice backgammon player, I could usually beat you 9 out of 10 times. And it wouldn't matter at all how the dice were rolling.

MY GREATEST MOMENT OF BACKGAMMON GLORY

Perhaps my greatest moment of backgammon glory came years ago when I was on vacation, by myself, in the Caribbean.

I was relaxing by the pool one day at the resort where I was staying. I had brought my backgammon set along with me and a nice young man from Brazil spotted it, so he approached me and asked if I'd like to play a game or two.

He turned out to be a pretty good backgammon player himself and we played several closely contested games, with each of us winning about equally.

Then, the most memorable backgammon victory I have ever engineered (or seen) took place.

In the final game that we played, I was so far behind that no one in their right mind would have given me even the slightest chance of winning. Only I was thinking just the opposite.

I was patiently biding my time, executing a carefully planned "reversal strategy" that could eventually turn the tables on my opponent. But I was running out of time.

My opponent had already gotten 14 of his 15 pieces safely off the board, and none of my 15 pieces was even close to coming off. His one remaining piece was just 4 spots away from the finish line, and he was clearly going to win the game on his very next roll, unless I managed to hit his one remaining piece with my upcoming roll, thereby sending it all the way back to the beginning.

This was the opportunity I had patiently been waiting for and that I had actually been planning for from the moment I got way behind.

Even though his one remaining piece was just 4 spots away from victory, I knew I had positioned most of my own pieces in good position to thwart him, by hitting his last piece and getting myself back in the game.

I also knew that I had positioned my pieces to have an excellent chance of "hitting" his one remaining piece, no matter what combination of dice I rolled on my very next throw.

So I confidently rolled the dice, hit his one remaining piece (as I believed I would), and then I managed to skillfully get all 15 of my pieces off the board before he could get his one single piece back in the game and around the board to safety!

Wow—that was a backgammon victory well worth remembering, savoring, and bragging about for a lifetime.

Now, I told you this story not simply to brag, but to impress upon you the magnitude of the incredible transformation I experienced. More importantly, I can now tell you about the one big secret I learned that made all the difference—both with regard to my being able to win at backgammon and then later on to being able to win against stress as well.

HOW I TURNED IT ALL AROUND

As you can see, in a very short time I went from knowing absolutely nothing about how to win at backgammon to knowing just a little, which was enough to make me a consistent loser. And then, some type of "miracle" occurred that enabled me to turn it all around and become an impressive, accomplished winner.

Well, the same thing happened with regard to my ability to win against stress. The very same life-mastery principle that enabled me to become a winner at backgammon also later enabled me to figure out how to become an equally impressive winner against stress.

This one key principle enabled me to finally gain greater personal control over my emotions, make dramatic improvements in my relationships, and achieve many other positive outcomes as well.

So what was it that made all the difference on that one magical day? What turned my life around back then as a backgammon player and later turned my whole life around as a stress sufferer? What major insight enabled me to not only figure out how to win at backgammon but also how to win the game of stress in my own life, and then go on to become a world-class expert?

SOMEONE HAD PITY ON ME!

What finally made the difference with regard to my losing at backgammon was that on that magical, life-changing day *someone had pity on me.* After watching me constantly lose and become frustrated time and time again, one of the two tennis pros (Jimmy) finally took me aside on that day and told me something I will never forget.

He said "I think you should go to the library and check out a few books about backgammon."

You have no idea how crazy this advice sounded to me. "You mean people have actually written books about backgammon?" I responded. I couldn't believe this was true. I knew people had written books about chess, but this was a much more complicated game. But writing books about backgammon? Come on, what is there to say about a game where you simply roll the dice and hope you get lucky?

But Jimmy assured me that people had indeed written books about backgammon and I should go read some of them. So I decided to take his advice. I went to my local library and sure enough there were books about backgammon there. I took a few of them home and started reading them.

Boy was my mind ever blown! I started learning about all sorts of cool strategies and principles for winning at backgammon that I never knew existed. And as I started to become aware of these hidden principles, I tested each of them out in simulated games, playing against myself, and I was amazed at how well they worked!

I then got additional books and set up my own individual training program. The more I practiced with the new concepts and strategies I was learning about, the more I could see improvements happening right on the board.

This is how I intentionally transformed myself from a consistent loser at backgammon to a very skillful and accomplished winner.

And here is the key life-mastery secret that made it all occur:

SECRET: The most important things you needed to know in order to become a top-notch winner at backgammon are all completely <u>invisible to the naked eye</u>!

The Invisible Game Of Backgammon

When I was consistently losing at backgammon, I had no idea that there were actually two games being played at the very same time. There was the *obvious game* of backgammon, where you roll the dice and move your pieces according to some easy to learn rules. And then there was the *invisible game* of backgammon, which I knew nothing about.

The invisible game was like a parallel universe, where those who knew about it became winners, and those who only played the obvious game got their money taken from them.

Without going into exhaustive detail—remember I told you this chapter is not about backgammon—let me share a few high-level things I learned about this invisible game that I never knew before.

Opening Move

Do you know that for every possible opening roll of the dice in backgammon, regardless of whether you go first or second, there is usually one best move for you to make? I didn't know that before, but it's true. And you can easily memorize these opening moves, once you understand why they are preferred.

Mid-Game Strategies

At any point in a backgammon game, you will either be ahead of your opponent, even with your opponent, or behind your opponent when it comes to advancing your 15 pieces toward the end goal of getting them all to safety and off the board.

Your position in relation to your opponent can change many times during each game. But whichever of these positions you find yourself in, there is one best strategy to adopt at any point in the game. If you are ahead, try to get even more ahead. If you are behind, don't try to catch up but get yourself "more behind" (I'll explain the wisdom of this in a moment). And if you are fairly even with your opponent, let it all hang out, take lots of risks, and go for broke. This way, you'll either get way ahead or way behind your opponent, and there are excellent strategies for winning from either of those two extreme positions.

Winning From Behind

Do you know that it's just as easy to win at backgammon when you are way behind as it is to win when you are way ahead?

This may sound unbelievable, but one of the cool things about backgammon is there are invisible strategies for winning from either position.

The invisible strategies for winning from behind are very different from the invisible strategies for winning when you're ahead. So you have to study them, practice them, and perfect them in order to consistently win with them. But my point is that once you truly understand the invisible game of backgammon, you can win most of the time *regardless of what the dice are doing.*

Protecting Your Assets

The obvious game of backgammon is all about rolls of the dice (yours and your opponent's) and hoping your exposed pieces (which you will inevitably have) don't get hit and sent back to the beginning.

The invisible game of backgammon, however, is not about hope or chance. It's about *mathematical probabilities*. There are only so many possible number combinations when two dice are rolled. And some of these combinations have greater mathematical probabilities of occurring than others. This is an important bit of knowledge to have at your fingertips.

Also, while there are 24 spaces (pointy triangle things) on a backgammon board, you may have choices during the game about where you are going to leave one of your pieces exposed, assuming you either want to or are forced to do this.

Knowing the best locations to leave your pieces exposed on the board, in relation to other pieces your opponent has positioned, is also a matter of mathematical probabilities. For example, any exposed piece of yours that is within six spaces of one of your opponent's pieces is mathematically much more likely to get hit than if it was seven spaces away or more.

Similar mathematical calculations also come into play with regard to where you position your groups of two or more pieces around the board. These groups of pieces effectively "block" your opponent from landing on those occupied spaces, so where you strategically locate these blockades can also make a big difference as to who ends up the victor.

The End Game

At the end of many backgammon games, both players will have most of their pieces grouped among the last six spaces on the board. Once all 15 of your pieces are within this final zone, you can then start taking them off the board, one or two at a time, depending upon each roll of the dice.

This can become a neck-and-neck race between two equally or nearly equally positioned opponents. So you have to be very strategic and maximally efficient with every single roll of the dice when you are within this "red zone" territory at the end of the game.

This becomes even more critical, since either you or your opponent could get lucky and roll "doubles," which could allow as many as 4 pieces to come off the board with just one turn. And since we don't want luck to ever determine the outcome, we really have to up our game in the red zone. Fortunately, there are a number of invisible strategies that can help you improve your odds.

THE INVISIBLE GAME OF STRESS

My purpose in writing this chapter is not to teach you how to win at backgammon—it's to show you something critically important that can help you become a winner against stress.

Just as with backgammon (and many other games or endeavors in life), if you don't know there's an invisible game going on, you are not going to fare as well as others who do know this invisible game exists and who have taken the time to learn how to master it.

And just as with backgammon, there is an *invisible game of stress* that most people have no idea is there and even fewer know how to win.

Step two in the Ultimate Method is all about how well (or not so well) you know how to play and win this invisible game.

In the next chapter, I'll shed some additional light on this invisible game of stress, including what it takes to become good at both playing and winning it.

CHAPTER 6: WHAT'S REALLY CAUSING YOUR STRESS TO OCCUR?

When it comes to understanding the true causes of our stress, what we see is not all there is. (Doc Orman, M.D.)

The greatest obstacle to discovery is not ignorance - it is the illusion of knowledge. (Daniel J. Boorstin)

I've already shown you how I applied one key life-mastery principle (the principle that what you see is not all there is) to consciously transforming myself into a winner at backgammon. In this chapter, I will show you how this very same principle can enable you to transform yourself into a consistent winner against stress.

YOU CAN LEARN TO WIN AGAINST STRESS

Just as with backgammon (and many other aspects of life), there is an *invisible game of stress* that most people have little awareness of and even fewer know how to master.

Those who do understand this invisible game, however, including its invisible rules, principles, and highly-effective strategies, are often much better able to deal with stress than others.

It's important to recognize that the specific rules, principles and strategies which underlie the invisible game of stress are vastly different from those that govern the game of backgammon. The only similarity is that *they are all entirely hidden from the untrained eye.*

Also, the invisible game of stress is much broader and more complex than backgammon. Thus, there are many more invisible rules, principles and strategies you will have to become aware of, given that stress comes in so many different forms and can arise from so many different sources and situations.

But while your task is larger and a bit more challenging, it is not impossible. It will take some work, commitment, and trial-and-error learning on your part. And it may also take some additional, more advanced training beyond what I can provide in this introductory level book.

But at least by the end of reading this book, you'll have a pretty good idea of what you need to do and what it takes to win.

My Own Personal Victory Over Stress

As I mentioned in the "Why I Wrote This Book" section, I may be an accomplished stress expert now, but for the first thirty years of my life I was absolutely terrible when it came to dealing with stress. I was tense, anxious, irritable, frustrated and angry much of the time. I had very little insight or control over my emotions, and I frequently was unhappy and even felt depressed fairly often.

Then I learned about the "what you see is not all there is" principle, and I began to apply it to many of the personal problems, emotional problems, and relationship problems I was having and that I had been struggling with unsuccessfully for years.

This led me down a new and different path that I had never explored before. And while it took me several years to become pretty good at understanding the invisible world of stress, I eventually gained many new insights and distinctions about this invisible world that enabled me to finally escape from being a perpetual loser to eventually becoming a consistent, accomplished winner.

MOST OF MY STRESS HAS BEEN GONE FOR YEARS

For the past 30 years of my life, even though I've had many more pressures and responsibilities than ever before, I've had very little stress or tension to speak of.

I rarely feel anxious, angry, or frustrated anymore, and even when I do, I know how to make those unwanted emotions quickly disappear whenever I want.

I've also been happily married to my wife Christina for 29 years, in addition to becoming one of the premier authors, educators, and stress coaches in the country today.

Don't make the mistake of thinking I was able to accomplish these changes because I possess certain talents or abilities that you might lack. It's entirely possible for anyone to duplicate the exact same success I had. In fact, it's even easier for you than it was for me, because I never had a book like this one, or like others that are available today, to guide me.

I OWE MY SUCCESS TO TWO THINGS

I owe most of this success at reducing stress in my life to two big things which I've already shared with you in this book:

1) The three-step Ultimate Method for dealing with any type of stress, and

2) My knowledge of specific internal causes of many different types of stress, which I have diligently accumulated over the years and which is absolutely essential for knowing how to execute each step (especially the second one) in this method properly.

Without having accumulated this stockpile of detailed, specific knowledge about the *invisible internal causes* that frequently contribute to our everyday stress, I too would be unable to get much value from attempting to use this method.

But once you know—in advance—what some of these common internal causes are, the game suddenly changes. Now you are in the driver's seat. Now you've suddenly got the upper hand over stress, even though stress may have been repeatedly kicking your butt before.

It's Like Playing A Hidden Picture Game

The process of spotting specific invisible, internal causes of your stress is very similar to playing a hidden picture game in a children's magazine.

You may recall these games where a complex drawing is presented to you with multiple hidden objects buried within the more obvious parts of the image. Right below the image, you see a list of hidden objects that you are challenged to find, like a spoon, a fireman's hat, a cow (usually upside down in a tree), a baseball bat, a hockey stick, etc.

With this helpful list in hand, you start looking at the picture again from different angles. All of a sudden, you are able to spot some of the hidden objects which had previously been invisible to you. One by one, you go through the list and if you stay with it long enough, you will eventually find all the hidden objects you didn't see initially.

Notice how useful that **list of hidden objects** was to your eventual success. Well, *the same is true for identifying the invisible causes of any stressful problem in life.*

It's very helpful to know—in advance—what those invisible causes are likely to be before you go searching for them deep within yourself. And when you know what some of these internal causes are, your ability to spot them (and complete step 2 of the Ultimate Method) will increase many fold.

EXAMPLES OF INTERNAL CAUSES OF STRESS

In order to complete step 2 of the Ultimate Method, you have to identify all of the major causes of any stressful problems you are experiencing. This means not only being able to recognize the obvious causes (usually external), but also being able to recognize invisible causes as well. These invisible, internal causes consist of thought patterns and/or behavior patterns **entirely within you**.

Now, you might be thinking there are an endless number of invisible, internal thought patterns and/or behavior patterns which can produce stress for human beings. And indeed, there are a great many of them. But becoming good at recognizing them is not as difficult as you might think.

This is because there's a reasonable number of hidden, internal causes (about a hundred of them) which are very common for all human beings. In addition, each person will have his or her own group of common, recurring internal causes. So once you learn how to identify these within yourself, you can pretty much count on them being involved, in one way or another, whenever you are feeling stressed.

I can't cover all hundred or so of these internal causes here in this introductory level book. But I can give you a few examples, just to show you that they aren't very difficult to understand. In fact, they often appear to be deceptively simple.

What makes these and other internal causes so difficult to spot is not their complexity—it's their *invisibility*! Since they occur entirely within us, they are often not readily apparent, especially when our attention is focused on external events, the behavior of others, and other external factors which may be contributing to our stress.

Here are six common internal causes that are frequently going to be lurking in the background (i.e., they will be mostly invisible) whenever you are experiencing any type of stress in your life. These six internal causes are:

Expectations

Good/Bad Thinking

Right/Wrong Thinking

Cause/Effect Thinking

Failing To Ask For Help

Failing To Admit You May Be Wrong

Think of this list as being just like the list of hidden objects in a hidden picture game. In other words, whenever you are feeling stressed, bring up this list and start searching for these six common internal causes within yourself. As with a hidden picture game, if you search long and hard enough, you'll probably find most of them playing an invisible role in whatever degree of stress you are feeling.

Let's now take a closer look at each of these six common internal causes.

NOTE: This is just a **starter list** of hidden, internal causes. There are many other internal causes that also might be playing a role in any type of stress you experience.

EXPECTATIONS

We all have internal expectations about a great many things. For instance, we have:

Expectations about ourselves

Expectations about other people

Expectations about life

Expectations about our cars

Expectations about our cell phones

Expectations about our computers

Expectations about our friends

Expectations about many other things.

Sometimes, we may be **consciously aware** of our internal expectations. Mostly, however, they exist in the **background** of our thinking and therefore they will be invisible to us.

Either way, expectations profoundly color our life, including how we react to everyday situations and events, and therefore how much stress we experience.

For example, many people have expectations that:

"Life should always be fair," or

"Friends should always be trustworthy."

When some random tragedy occurs, or if a long-time friend suddenly betrays them, their unseen expectations kick in and make an unfortunate situation feel even worse.

Tragedies and **betrayals** are the obvious causes that are clearly apparent to the stressed individual.

Internal expectations, on the other hand, are usually hidden from their view. This is why the role these internal factors play in causing stress in our lives is frequently missed.

Expectations frequently cause us to experience many types of stress, including:

Emotional distress

Relationship conflicts

Communication breakdowns

Work-related stress

School-related stress

And much more.

NOTE: The more you become aware of your hidden expectations, the more you will be able to use the third step in the Ultimate Method to start exerting more direct personal control over them.

GOOD/BAD THINKING

Another frequent hidden cause of human stress is our tendency to think in **Either/Or** terms. There are many variations on this theme, and I've included three of them in your starter list of six common internal causes.

Good/Bad thinking means that when certain things happen, we tend to automatically judge them to be either "good" or "bad."

For example:

Traffic jams are "bad." Courteous drivers are "good."

Being honest is "good." Being dishonest is "bad."

The problem with all types of automatic, either/or thinking is that they create false, mutually exclusive conceptual dichotomies that we tend to mistake for truths. In other words, we tend to automatically get stuck in just one side of an either/or dichotomy. This makes it difficult to appreciate additional, legitimate aspects of reality that belong to the opposite side.

Consider the following example:

You wake up one morning and discover your car has been stolen. This sudden realization is likely to automatically trigger negative internal thoughts within you, such as:

"This is really bad."

"My plans for today are totally ruined."

As a direct result of these automatic negative thoughts, you may experience strong negative emotions, such as sadness, anger, anxiety, or worry.

Now the point of this example is not to suggest you should consider having your car stolen a "good" thing. That would be silly.

Rather, it's to highlight how easily we automatically get stuck in just the "bad" side of this Good/Bad dichotomy. This then causes us to react to events exclusively in a **negative way**.

There are several problems with **Good/Bad Thinking** that we fail to appreciate when trying to correctly understand the causes of our stress. The first is that we generally don't recognize that we are engaging in either/or thinking (i.e., this is invisible to us). In addition, we fail to appreciate that the events that happen in our lives and our internal assessments of **good** or **bad** are two entirely separate things.

Events happen either inside or outside our bodies. But assessments are added separately by us internally (another process that's usually invisible to us). Thus, we end up mistakenly thinking that whatever happened really was inherently good or bad. This means we end up believing that "goodness" and "badness" are qualities of events themselves—and not internal judgments we either consciously or unconsciously attach to events.

The Truth about Good and Bad

Events in life are never inherently good or bad. They only become "good" or "bad" when human beings add these interpretations to them.

In addition, few events in life deserve to be interpreted as either entirely good or entirely bad. Most events usually have both good **and** bad aspects to them, depending on how we choose to relate to them and what we choose to focus upon. Also, we can choose to respond to most events in life in ways that can produce either positive or negative outcomes (or both).

So, if you automatically tend to focus on just the bad side of a good/bad dichotomy, you may become "blind" to any **positive benefits** that could also be involved. And if you tend to focus on just the good side, you may miss **potential risks** or other important **negatives**.

Right/Wrong Thinking

Another common either/or pattern that causes a great deal of human stress is **Right/Wrong thinking**.

Right/Wrong thinking describes our tendency to judge our own or others' behaviors as being either totally "right" or totally "wrong."

Throughout human history, many adverse consequences (and stress) have emerged from Right/Wrong thinking. For example, almost every war ever fought came from Right/Wrong thinking. And when it comes to marital problems, divorces, and other interpersonal conflicts, Right/Wrong thinking is commonly involved.

Again, the problem with this way of thinking and all other forms of either/or thinking, is two-fold: 1) we get trapped into thinking that the **truth** is one-sided, with people being either completely right or completely wrong; and 2) we are usually not aware that Right/Wrong thinking has taken us over.

This makes it difficult to appreciate just how often we draw false conclusions about other people, devalue their legitimate opinions, or misinterpret their actual motives and intentions.

NOTE: Right/Wrong thinking and Good/Bad thinking are frequently involved as invisible, internal causes of our **negative emotions**, such as anger, guilt, fear, worry, and frustration. So whenever you are experiencing any strong negative emotion, always look for one or both of these internal causes playing a major role. Then, if you spot these hidden culprits, you can use the third step in the Ultimate Method to make most negative emotions (and many other types of stress) naturally disappear whenever you want.

Cause/Effect Thinking

Another either/or pattern of thinking that gets us into trouble (and also produces stress) is Cause/Effect thinking. When we engage in this type of thinking, we typically assume that whatever happens in life comes from linear, sequential cause-effect dynamics.

Unfortunately, real life doesn't usually happen in linear causal ways. Real life mostly happens through complex, multi-dimensional causes.

For example, when something goes wrong, it is rarely because one person or one single factor was responsible. Usually, there are multiple causal factors involved, but we don't see all of these multiple factors clearly because we've been trained to think in simplistic, linear ways.

One common consequence of linear causal thinking is that we tend to blame people (including ourselves) for things that turn out poorly, as if there was only one causative agent involved. Once again, this is rarely the case. And our blame, therefore, is often too narrowly placed.

Another area where cause/effect thinking leads us to draw many false conclusions is our understanding of health and human illness. We have many cause/effect theories about what makes people sick and also what keeps us well. Unfortunately, many of these theories are either wholly or partially wrong. This can lead to unnecessary stress in many different ways, which are far too complex to delve into here.

FAILING TO ASK FOR HELP

A very common *action pattern* that frequently leads to much human stress is **Failing To Ask For Help**.

As we go through life, we often encounter problems that could be solved or avoided if we just sought help from others. Unfortunately, we have many internal barriers that keep us from doing this.

For example, we have internal thought barriers like:

"I should always solve my problems on my own."

"Asking for help is a sign of weakness."

"If I ask for help, others might think I'm stupid."

"I'm much too embarrassed to ask for assistance."

"I don't want to burden other people."

"I asked for help in the past and it didn't work out."

We also have barriers in the form of internal action patterns, such as:

Procrastination

Being unwilling to pay for expert help

Not being open to good, sound advice from others.

Again, **Failing To Ask For Help** is a very common action pattern (within us) that frequently leads to stress. Unfortunately, this common factor often goes unrecognized as a common internal cause of many of our stressful problems in life.

FAILING TO ADMIT YOU MAY BE WRONG
Here's an internal *action pattern* that's goes hand-in-hand with an internal *thought pattern*—both of which combine to produce a powerful tandem cause of human stress.

As I've already pointed out, Right/Wrong thinking and other types of either/or thinking often lead to errors in judgment or errors in perception. When this happens, we tend to compound things further because we are often reluctant to admit (or even consider) that we may be wrong.

It's kind of a double whammy or 1-2 punch, where two invisible factors take hold of us and keep us from: 1) recognizing what is really going on, and 2) making needed corrections that could help us reduce our stress.

DETAILED KNOWLEDGE ABOUT SPECIFIC INTERNAL CAUSES

Remember, these are only six of many common internal causes of human stress. But this is the type of detailed, specific knowledge you'll need to have at your fingertips if you want to be able to use the Ultimate Method successfully.

As I said at the outset, this three-step method is not quite as easy as it looks. There's much detailed knowledge you'll need to acquire to make it work, given that stress can come in hundreds of different forms.

But once you get good at recognizing some of the common internal thought patterns and behavior patterns that typically arise for you, you'll begin spotting these everywhere. Regardless of what specific type of stress you may be experiencing—be it emotional stress, stress at work, stress at school, family stress, financial stress, the stress of public speaking, the stress of dealing with serious illness, etc.—many of these same internal causes are going to be involved most of the time.

So how can you benefit from accurately pinpointing these six specific internal causes? How does this help you prevent or eliminate stress without having to use drugs, relaxation exercises or other time-consuming stress management techniques?

The real benefit comes when you know how to apply the third and final step in the Ultimate Method. In the next chapter, I will show you what it takes to do this.

SPECIAL NOTE: If you'd like to receive a list of the 65 internal causes of stress I discuss in my book *The 14 Day Stress Cure*, just go to www.theultimatemethod.com where you can download this list for free. It's only a two page list that gives you just the names of these 65 internal causes, without explanations, but it's still a very handy list to have, because it can give you some direction when you are feeling stressed and you are interested in identifying internal causes.

Chapter 7: How To Make Stress Quickly Disappear

There is one thing even more vital to science than intelligent methods; and that is, the sincere desire to find out the truth, whatever it may be. (Charles Pierce)

Most people assume there are only three things you can do about stressful negative emotions, such as anger, frustration, etc.:

You can *express* them (by yelling, screaming, or punching things)

You can *suppress* them (and run the risk of making yourself sick)

You can *manage* them (taking deep breaths, journaling, exercising regularly, meditating, etc.)

There's actually a fourth way to deal with negative emotions—you can make them quickly and naturally *disappear* by correctly applying the third step in the Ultimate Method. And this is not limited to emotional stress alone. You can do the very same thing with other types of stress as well.

You've Already Done This!

You may not be aware of this fourth possibility, but you've already experienced it.

Here's one example: Say you made arrangements with a friend to meet you at an agreed upon place and time for a very important reason. Say you needed them to transport you somewhere, and if they didn't show up you were going to miss out on a big opportunity. And let's assume that you clearly communicated to your friend the importance of not forgetting to be there and of being on time.

When your big day comes, you make sure to arrive at the meeting place way ahead of time. But when it's time for your friend to meet you...no one shows up. You decide to give them a few extra minutes, but you're feeling a little peeved that they didn't arrive on time.

Ten more minutes go by and your friend is still not there. Now you are really pissed. Ten more minutes go by and you transition to full-blown anger.

Why were you feeling so angry? Well, you've probably judged your friend to be irresponsible, lazy, unreliable, untrustworthy, forgetful or something else like that. You've certainly assumed that they didn't take being on time as seriously as you thought they should.

Then, all of a sudden your friend arrives, looking harried and stressed as well. They inform you they left their house early to meet you, but they ran into an unexpected traffic jam that they couldn't escape from. They are extremely apologetic and you realize this is one of those things that can happen to anyone, through no neglectful fault of their own.

Now here's the key point of this example: What happened to your anger the moment you discovered the truth about what really happened? It *instantly disappeared*, didn't it? Your anger vanished in a flash, quickly and naturally, without you having to do anything at all to deal with it! One minute you were feeling extremely angry, and the next minute—poof— all your anger was instantly gone.

What caused this sudden disappearance of your anger to occur? You might think it was simply finding out the truth about what really happened, and you would be partly correct. But that wasn't the whole story. There was another process that took place deep within you, only you didn't notice this change because it was *invisible*. But it took place nonetheless, else your anger would not have gone away.

Internal "Realities"

One of the ways the invisible game of stress gets played is this: The internal thought patterns and behavior patterns that contribute to our stress do so by creating all sorts of internal "realities" within us. Sometimes these internal realities are true or useful...and sometimes they are not.

Either way, our bodies don't know the difference.

Our bodies assume that all of our internal "realities" are *absolutely true.* This is where our emotions (and other types of stress) come from, whether we are aware of these invisible processes going on in our bodies or not.

In the example above, you originally became angry because when your friend didn't arrive on time, this triggered certain thought patterns and behavior patterns that created an internal "reality" in your body. This internal "reality" was that your friend had acted irresponsibly, neglectfully, or otherwise inappropriately. This was a false internal "reality" right from the get go, but both you and your body didn't know this at the time. Hence you reacted with anger because a specific internal "reality" got triggered within you, and because both you and your body automatically assumed that it was true.

But when your friend arrived and told you what really happened, your false internal "reality" got shattered and could no longer be maintained. It disintegrated instantly, deep within in your body, and your anger vanished with it, because the key invisible force that was driving your angry feelings could no longer be viewed as valid.

WHAT CAN WE LEARN FROM THIS EXAMPLE?

There's a great deal we can learn from this very common example, which almost everyone has experienced. The first is that feelings of anger (and many other types of stress) can and do instantly disappear. This can occur when we recognize that one or more of our internal "realities" are not really true.

The second thing to take away from this example is to appreciate that this is not an isolated, uncommon occurrence for human beings. There are countless other events in life that trigger false internal "realities" within us all the time. In fact, this happens to each of us multiple times every day! But this all goes on *invisibly*, so we don't notice how often it occurs.

A third thing you can gain from this example is that you don't necessarily have to depend upon good fortune or luck to discover that one of your triggered, internal "realities" is not entirely valid. In the example above, your friend eventually showed up and provided you with the correct information. Had they never arrived, you would still likely be angry.

But you don't have to wait for someone else or for future life events to show you that you were wrong. You can do this yourself, whenever you want. Once you recognize that a specific thought pattern or behavior pattern is contributing to your stress, you can decide to question its validity anytime you choose. You can become your own *false internal "reality" detector* and help yourself eliminate many types of stress, quickly and easily, by doing so.

Of course, another part of the invisible game of stress is that you will have to do battle with another formidable internal opponent that we've already talked about—Failing To Admit You May Be Wrong—before you can get good at doing this. But this barrier to winning the game of stress can be overcome if you are serious enough about wanting to surmount it.

THE AWESOME POWER OF DISCONFIRMATION

Lots of people talk about personal empowerment today, and even more talk about self-improvement and personal growth. But I know of few things more self-empowering for any human being than developing the fine art of self-directed disconfirmation.

Disconfirmation is a powerful coping strategy that cognitive psychologists highlighted many years ago. It's simply the act of intentionally trying to "disconfirm" particular thoughts, ideas, and perceptions that commonly arise within you but that may not be either useful or true.

As I mentioned before, our bodies tend to automatically assume that most of our internal thoughts and perceptions are absolutely true (and therefore our associated feelings are valid). These assumptions about the world may never have been rigorously tested, but that doesn't matter. As far as our bodies are concerned, they are assumed to be true until proven otherwise.

So we often go through life accumulating many false ideas that we believe to be true but that are either partly or entirely incorrect. *And these false ideas are very frequent contributors to much of the stress we experience.*

This is another important aspect of the invisible game of stress that most people never appreciate. In many ways, it's very similar to how I was completely unaware of the invisible game of backgammon, even though this game was actually there all along, and its dynamics had been operating invisibly for thousands of years!

The Third Step In The Ultimate Method

So the third step in the Ultimate Method is to try to actively "disconfirm" any thought patterns or behavior patterns that you correctly identify as contributing to your stress in step 2 of the Method.

Note that as long as you remain completely unaware of the hidden, internal causes producing stress within you, there's little you can do to combat them. On the other hand, once you become aware of them (step 2), you now have many new options available to you.

For example, when we automatically view something as "bad" (Good/Bad thinking), we can mistakenly assume that whatever happened **really was bad**, and therefore there is little good that can come from it.

This can lead to unnecessary stress in our lives, because the truth about life is often very different from the internal "realities" that get triggered within us.

But once you are aware that you've fallen into a "Good/Bad" pattern of thinking and that this specific pattern often leads to distorted, inaccurate internal "realities," you have options and choices that may not have been available to you before.

For instance, you could now:

Remind yourself that events and your interpretation of those events are two entirely separate things;

Consciously choose how you are going to interpret your situation. In other words, are you going to continue viewing life from your automatic "bad" perspective (once you become aware of it), or are you going to open your mind to other ways of looking at your situation?

Let's go back to the example of your car being stolen, which we discussed in the previous chapter.

Discovering that your car has been stolen may instantly trigger you to feel "bad" because you automatically judged your predicament from a negative "either/or" perspective.

It may seem that the event itself (losing your car) is inherently bad—but this is an illusion. In reality, two things actually happened:

The event—losing your car, and

Your automatic interpretation that this event is "bad."

But once you move this formerly invisible process—judging events as being "bad"—out into the open, you can now honestly evaluate your interpretations and seek to disconfirm any that may not be totally true.

By making this key distinction, which is something we all have the power to do, you suddenly become free to choose other ways of looking at your situation. You may even find there are other, more useful stress-relieving perspectives that can make you feel better or allow you to cope with your situation much more easily or creatively.

CHOOSE HOW YOU WANT TO VIEW EVENTS

When you become consciously aware that external events and your internal assessments (such as "good" and "bad") are separate things, you don't have to remain stuck in your automatic, triggered "either/or" viewpoints.

You can begin to see beyond the limits of these narrow, internal perspectives, and you can consciously choose whether you want to continue with them, or not:

Here are a few questions you would then be free to explore:

What if losing your car isn't quite as bad as you originally thought?
Are there any good things that might result from this?
Is there any way you can turn this loss into something positive?
What else could you do to creatively keep this event from ruining your day?

Again, don't get me wrong here. I'm not saying you should view losing your car as a "good" thing or that you should never, ever view it as something "bad."

I am simply trying to point out that as human beings, we commonly fail to appreciate how often our emotional and behavioral responses to certain events in life, such as losing one's car, are caused in part by internal thought patterns and internal behavior patterns that are often completely invisible to us.

The more our automatic perspectives and internal "realities" deviate from true reality, the more problems we will encounter in life, and therefore the more stress we will have.

REALISTICALLY EVALUATE YOUR HIDDEN EXPECTATIONS

The same process of self-directed disconfirmation can be applied to virtually any kind of stress, once you correctly pinpoint its internal causes. For instance, it can be applied to any of your internal expectations, once you recognize them. As you become more aware of specific internal expectations that may be contributing to your stress, you can use this third step in the Ultimate Method to free yourself from them.

This may sound overly simplistic, but it's true nonetheless. However, it's one thing to become aware of your internal expectations and quite another to know which ones are realistic and which ones aren't. This is a challenge, but it can be met.

For example, if you notice you have the specific expectation "Life should always be fair," you could stop and ask yourself: "Is this really true?"

By consciously reflecting upon this one expectation, you may be able to discover flaws in its logic.

The same can be done with all "either/or" patterns of thinking, once you become aware of them.

Is it true that whatever someone did or said was totally **right** or totally **wrong**?

Are your cause/effect theories well informed and accurate, or are they either partly or entirely misleading?

You'd be surprised how often your conclusions might change, once you ask yourself these very simple disconfirming questions. And this is the secret to knowing how to win the invisible game of stress by knowing how to make stress naturally disappear without having to manage it.

CHAPTER 8: WHY MANAGE YOUR STRESS WHEN YOU CAN BANISH IT INSTEAD?

Alice came to a fork in the road. 'Which road do I take?' she asked. 'Where do you want to go?' responded the Cheshire Cat. 'I don't know,' Alice answered. 'Then,' said the Cat, 'it doesn't matter.' (Lewis Carroll)

'As much money and life as you could want!'—the two things most human beings would choose above all. The trouble is, humans do have a knack of choosing precisely those things that are worst for them." (J.K. Rowling)

You've now been introduced to the Ultimate Method for dealing with stress and have seen that when used correctly, it can be much more powerful and versatile than stress management.

You've also seen that it's humanly possible to make certain types of stress quickly disappear by identifying underlying causes (both external and internal) and then by acting to correct (disconfirm) any internal causes (within you) that may be erroneous.

So how can you get to the point where you can use this Method consistently and successfully? How can you truly become an accomplished winner at both playing and winning the invisible game of stress?

BECOME A STUDENT OF INTERNAL CAUSES

The best way to do this is to become a perpetual student of internal causes. If you adopt the philosophy that every stressful problem in life always has both external and internal causes, then there are literally hundreds and hundreds of internal causes of stress you might want to learn more about.

The more you become familiar with some of these typical internal causes, the better you will become at using the Ultimate Method successfully.

For instance:

How well do you understand the internal causes of anger, guilt, frustration, fear, worry, sadness and other negative emotions?

Can you name the top ten internal causes of relationship stress and relationship failures?

How about the top ten internal causes of work related stress, or school related stress or the fear of public speaking?

Do you know the leading internal causes of holiday stress, which usually starts around November for many people and lasts through the end of each year?

Or how about the internal causes of financial stress, panic attacks, test anxiety, low self-esteem, lack of joy and happiness, fear of crowds, fear of snakes, or fear of spiders?

I could keep listing additional stressful problems, but I think you get the point. The more you know about hidden, internal causes of specific problems in life, the better you will become at solving these problems by attacking their causes, rather than endlessly spinning your wheels trying to deal with just their symptoms alone.

So if you don't know the answers to each of the questions I posed above, how can you acquire these answers? What steps can you take, once you finish reading this book, to continue exploring the internal causes of many types of stress so you can become better and better at spotting them and then using the Ultimate Method to defeat them?

GET SOME ADDITIONAL TRAINING

The best way to gain this type of stress-relieving knowledge is to get some additional training. Remember, the biggest challenge with expanding your awareness of internal causes is that they are mostly invisible to the untrained eye.

Sure you can try to identify them on your own, but this is the hard way to go. Better to seek help from others who have already figured out some of these internal causes and who are willing to share their knowledge with you.

One way to do this is to read books on different subjects written by highly qualified experts. Recall that this is exactly what I did to learn how to first understand and then master the hidden dynamics of backgammon.

But I've also read many books about cognitive psychology, happiness, self-improvement, family dynamics, relationship skills, communications skills, writing skills, computer skills, marketing strategies, and a whole bunch of other subjects. And obviously, as a physician, I've read and continue to read a number of sources of high quality information about health, illness, wellness and human well-being.

So you can set up a very nice training program for yourself, just by finding a bunch of high-quality books and studying them diligently. You might want to start off with some of my other Kindle books about stress, if any of those topics interest you.

ATTEND LIVE WORKSHOPS AND SEMINARS

Another good way to keep expanding your awareness of internal causes is to attend high-quality interactive workshops and seminars. These are available on a wide array of topics all throughout the U.S. and even internationally.

I've gained a good bit of my knowledge about internal causes by attending such live training events. I've also delivered hundreds of live training programs myself, which were designed to impart this same type of stress relief wisdom to all who participated.

ASSOCIATE WITH OTHER PEOPLE WHO SHARE YOUR SAME GOAL

Another powerful way to expand your knowledge of the hidden, internal causes of stress is to hang out with other people who are interested in this very same goal. With all the many online forums, local support groups, local Meetups, and groups on Facebook, LinkedIn, Google Plus and elsewhere, I'm sure you can find groups that might already be doing this, or you could start a group of your own. For example, you could invite people to get a copy of this book, read it, and then come together to help each other become better at using the Ultimate Method.

I am also developing an international community of like-minded people who are interested in achieving higher levels of stress reduction than stress management can provide. These are people—like yourself—who have already been exposed to the Ultimate Method and who are hungry to learn more about how to use it expertly.

I am building this community through my Stress Mastery Academy, and you are welcome to join us if you'd like. The cost is a one-time fee of less than $10, and this includes an excellent advanced training course on the Ultimate Method, along with a subscription to our 52-week email newsletter.

You can find out more about how to join this Academy by going to www.stressmasteryacademy.com and downloading the free special report pictured below:

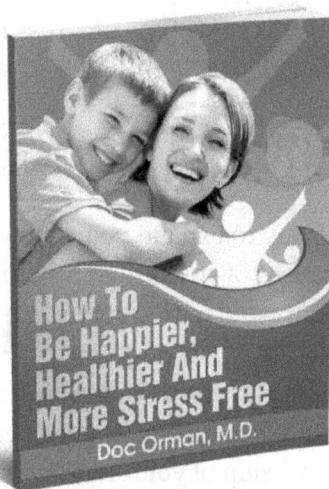

At the end of this report, you'll learn all about the Academy and the four e-book course you'll receive when you join. This is the advanced training course on the Ultimate Method that I mentioned above. It covers many of the same points revealed in this book, but it also goes into much more detail about internal causes and gives you many more examples. It would be an excellent next step for you if you liked what you learned here and want to get some additional, more advanced training.

Also, when you visit this website, you'll see a tab labeled "Video Lesson." When you click on this tab, you can watch a ten minute video lesson where I talk about and reveal the hidden causes of anger.

If you already know that you want to join the Academy, you can bypass the free report and go directly to www.stressmasteryacademy.com/join.

PRACTICE UNTIL YOU GET REALLY GOOD

However you decide to go about expanding your knowledge of internal causes and improving your ability to benefit from the Ultimate Method, you'll need to practice and then practice again until you get really good at using this method.

Remember, in order to use the Ultimate Method successfully, you must get good at several key skills. These include:

Letting go of your habit of calling your problems "stress"

Defining your true problems specifically and accurately

Identifying specific internal causes

Dealing effectively with internal causes until your stressful problems lessen or completely disappear.

Each of these skills requires practice, patience and repetition. And remember, since the key internal causes of your stressful problems in life are not going to be visible to you, you will have to work at learning how to spot their telltale signs in many different situations.

IT GETS EASIER AS TIME GOES ON

The good news is that the more you work at developing your new stress mastery skills, the easier this becomes as time goes on. After a while, the knowledge and skills you acquire will become second nature to you, so you won't have to work at recalling them. You'll just naturally go through life, and these insights will be there for you to effortlessly draw upon anytime you might need them.

So why would you want to keep managing your stress when you can learn how to simply banish it instead? "I guess it all depends on what you want," said the cat...with a grin.

CONCLUSION

In conclusion, I hope you've enjoyed learning about the Ultimate Method and how it can benefit you. You have enough general knowledge now that you can go out and start experimenting with this method immediately.

However, don't expect to make most types of stress in your life immediately disappear by trying to apply this method initially. That would be an unrealistic expectation which could cause you stress. But you might be able to have some successes right away and then more over time, as you get more experience with the method and continue to expand your skills.

Also, if you enjoyed reading this book, I encourage you to go back and read both of the first two books in this series:

Stress Relief Wisdom: Ten Key Distinctions For A Stress Free Life

The Choice Of Paradox: How "Opposite Thinking" Can Improve Your Life And Reduce Your Stress

These two books will help you better understand some of the deeper philosophies that underlie this powerful approach to dealing with stress, as well as giving you some additional training and insights that can help you right away.

Thanks for taking the time to learn about the Ultimate Method, and I hope you will find it more and more helpful as time goes on.

I look forward to sharing even more secrets about relieving stress with you in the very near future.

To your health, happiness, and success,

Doc Orman, M.D.

About The Author

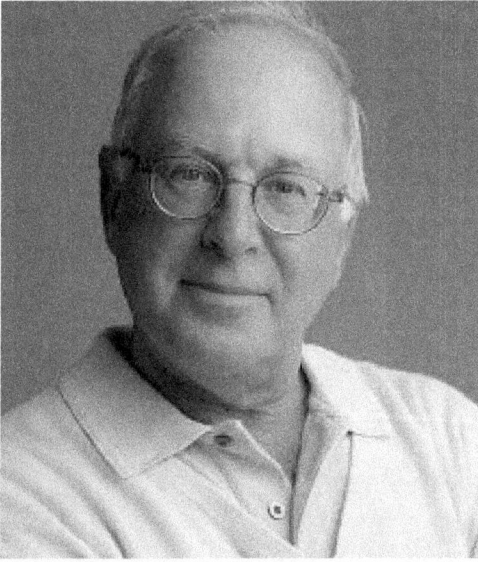

MORT (Doc) ORMAN, M.D. is an Internal Medicine physician, author, stress coach, and founder of the Stress Mastery Academy. He has been teaching people how to eliminate stress, without managing it, for more than 30 years. He has also conducted seminars and workshops on reducing stress for doctors, nurses, veterinarians, business executives, students, the clergy, and even the F.B.I. Dr. Orman's award-winning book, The 14 Day Stress Cure (1991), is still one of the most helpful and innovative books on the subject of stress ever written. Dr. Orman and his wife, Christina, a veterinarian, live in Maryland.

* 9 7 8 1 6 3 1 6 1 0 0 9 7 *